SERMONS
Part II

SERMONS
Part II

Melissa J. Weeks-Richardson

Library of Congress Control Number: 2022921473
ISBN: Hardcover   978-1-6698-5566-8
                 Softcover   978-1-6698-5565-1
                 eBook   978-1-6698-5564-4

Print information available on the last page.

Rev. date: 11/11/2022

To order additional copies of this book, contact:
Xlibris
844-714-8691
www.Xlibris.com
Orders@Xlibris.com
847963

Contents

Preface vii

"The Joy of the Lord Is Your Strength" 1

"Be Anxious for Nothing" 3

"Jesus Says, 'Take Me at My Word'" 5

"Forgiveness" 8

"Take It to the Lord in Prayer" 14

"Lord, Teach Us" 17

"Nevertheless" 19

"A Psalm of Deliverance" 21

"God Is Light" 23

"Destined to Win" 26

"Touch Not My Anointed and Do My Prophet No Harm" 30

"It Rains on the Just and the Unjust" 34

"Saving the Best for Last" 39

"If I Be Lifted Up" 42

A Mother's Love 46

"Get Your House in Order for Jesus Is Soon to Come Back" 48

And His Name Shall Be Called Jesus 51

Sources 55

Author's Publications 57

Author's Songs 59

Index 61

Preface

Sermons Part II is just a few of my many sermons that that God allowed to preach over the last fifteen years. There are often times I find myself looking and listening to other sermons—at times, for encouragement or, sometimes, just because I have been inspired by certain preachers. These sermons are to inspire, uplift, encourage, guide, and correct. These transforming messages have been put together to impact lives globally.

TITLE: *"The Joy of the Lord Is Your Strength"*

TEXT: Nehemiah 8:9–10 KJV

AUTHOR: Nehemiah or Ezra or perhaps both

DATE AND PLACE: Written in Palestine 446–430 BC, sometime after the second trip of Nehemiah to Jerusalem in the thirty-second year of Artaxerxes.

The scripture begins with the people gathering themselves together as one man into the street (this being described as a broad, open space). It mentions before the water gate. The water gate was located near the Gihon Spring on the east side of Jerusalem.

Here, the Bible states that they spake unto Ezra the Scribe to bring the book of the Law of Moses, which the Lord had commanded to Israel.

First, they requested Ezra to bring the book of the Law of Moses. I must remind you, this is still God's law. Second, Ezra was going to teach the people these laws.

How do we know that Ezra was going to teach the people these laws? This is the first mention of Ezra in the book of Nehemiah. When you look back, Nehemiah had been ministering in Jerusalem as far back as 458 BC.

We can also gain from the text that Ezra was a priest as well as a scribe. Who were scribes? Scribes studied the law. The priest's duty was and still is to teach people the Word of God. Reading and explaining the scripture took place from morning until midday. This was about six hours. Nehemiah was not only a cupbearer, but he also served as governor at the time of reading the law.

When the people heard the words of the law and began to understand, they began to weep. However, this weeping was out of repentance. They were instructed to turn their weeping into rejoicing—to go their way, eat the fat, drink the sweet, and send portions unto those whom nothing is prepared. Why, because this day is holy for our Lord. For the joy of the Lord is your strength.

That day was a holy day of worship, preparing them for what was to come. There would be hard days ahead, but the joy of the Lord would be their strength. The joy of the Lord is your strength.

No matter how hard things may seem, the joy of the Lord is your strength. Keep pushing. Knowing that with God on your side, you can make it. I know you feel like throwing in the towel, but there is joy in knowing that the Lord is sustaining you enough to keep you going. The joy of knowing that the Lord fights your battle is enough to keep you going. The joy of knowing that He walks with me (you), and He talks with me (you), and that He tells me (you) that I (you) am (are) His own is sustaining. No matter how things look around you, no matter how you feel, just know that the joy of the Lord is your strength.

TITLE: *"Be Anxious for Nothing"*
SUBTOPIC: "Being Grateful in the Time of a Pandemic"
TEXT: Philippians 4:6 NKJV
AUTHOR: Paul
DATE AND PLACE: Written from Rome about AD 64
THEME: The joy of Christian grace and experience in all of life and death

----

The word translated as "be anxious" in Philippians 4:6 is *merimnao.* Using the Greek English Lexicon of New Testament and early Christian literature, there are several translations of merimnao: "to have anxiety" or to be "unduly concerned." It is referring to worry.

There are times in our lives when we all have faced times when we have worried about certain issues. It may have been a family issue, a health issue, a financial issue, or about some sort of issue that we have no control over. Paul's advice is to turn our worries into praise.

Paul here is telling believers to avoid anxiety and worry. We have to trust God with our needs and have a grateful attitude. Paul is encouraging prayer and supplication with thanksgiving.

The Bible tells us in verse 6 to be anxious for nothing. It also talks about how one's life can be from sinful fretting. Everything should be taken to the Lord in prayer—everything from wayward children, health issues, lonely feelings, marital problems, mental health issues, to financial issues. There is nothing too great or too small for God's hands to hold.

During the holiday seasons of 2020, we experienced something new. This year, we are celebrating the holidays all over the world while experiencing a pandemic. Hundreds of thousands of people have lost their lives. This means that many have lost their loved ones. The unemployment rate is high because many have lost their jobs and many have lost their homes.

Many have had to do things that they have never had to do before, such as rely on food banks to sustain them, and at the same time, they would like to provide Christmas gifts for their families.

Let me encourage you to hold your head up and be grateful in a time of a pandemic and remind you that all is not lost. If God has allowed you to hear my voice or to read this book, you have something to be grateful for. I do not know all that God has allowed you to go through. However, I do know that if you still have breath in your body, that is enough to be grateful for.

I know that you may not have everything you want; however, if you still have lights, running water, and a roof over your head, that is enough to be grateful. If your bills are paid, sure, you may not be able to do everything you did last year, and sure, people may talk about you, but whom are you trying to please? That is enough to be grateful for.

Somewhere down the line, we have forgotten the simple things that God have allowed us to be able to enjoy in life, such as being able to heat our homes, being able to enjoy the pleasure of sleeping in a nice, comfortable bed at night, being able to take a warm shower, and being able to drink a glass of cold water. Let us be grateful for those things this season. Let us thank God for the little things and remind Him of how we appreciate them.

There is somebody. If you were to call their name, they would not be able to answer. There is somebody that is praying and hoping that they can take a warm shower. There is somebody that cannot remember that last time they had a hot bowl of soup.

The next time you want to complain about what you do not have control over or what you do not have, remember, there is someone that is worse off than you are, and that if somebody else was dealt the cards that you were dealt, they would play it very well.

Prayer is both an act and an atmosphere. We come to the Lord at specific times and bring specific requests before Him. It is also possible to live in an atmosphere of prayer.

The mood of our life should be a prayerful mood. Prayer in this verse signifies the overall attitude. Supplication signifies specific requests, which we bring to the Lord. However, requests should be made known to God with thanksgiving. In other words, you need to be anxious in nothing, prayerful in everything, and thankful for anything. Whenever you start to worry, take a moment, stop, and pray.

TITLE: *"Jesus Says, 'Take Me at My Word'"*

TEXT: John 4:46–54

AUTHOR: John

DATE AND PLACE: Written in about AD 90 in a place unknown

Historical Background

The scripture text is centered on Jesus healing an official's son. This official was of royal status. According to Finis Dake, he was an officer or perhaps a prince. Some scholars pointed out that he was one of the royal family or an officer of Herod Antipas, tetrarch of Galilee, as noted in Luke 3:1 and Matthew 14:1. Here we see Jesus visited Cana in Galilee. This is the place where Jesus was on the third day after He left Jordan to start his ministry (John 2:1). This was also the place where Jesus turned water into wine.

Here we see that Jesus was approached by the nobleman or royal official who was from Capernaum. This official had a son who was sick back in Capernaum. We also see that two things took place. The first thing that took place is, we see that the parent seeks Christ. Second, we see the parent intercedes on behalf of the child.

I know you are wondering where that came from. Well, let us go back over it. Verse 47 said that when the nobleman heard that Jesus had come out of Judaea into Galilee, he went unto Him and besought Him that He would come down and heal his son for he was at the point of death.

According to the *Strong's Expanded Concordance*, the Greek word for *besought*, as explained, is *erotao*, which means to "request, ask, beseech, pray, desire, or entreat." It is used by a king in making a request from another king (Luke 14:32).

So now, you see where several events took place. First, the nobleman or official went to Jesus. This man was a parent first, and then he was a man of royal status second. This was a man who has the authority to send people to come to him. However, this royal official, this man of royal status, humbled himself instead. He knew who Jesus was. He knew that Jesus had what he needed. Regardless of his royal status, there was still something that he could not obtain without going to Jesus.

Second, this royal official went to Jesus. Going to Jesus required him to be in His presence. This means that he had to come before Jesus. He was seeking Jesus. Remember, Jesus was not seeking him. When he heard Jesus had come out of Judaea into Galilee, he went unto Him because he had to seek Him.

Are you seeking Him?

Finally, he begged Jesus to come and heal his son. This means that some communication had to take place. The nobleman had to open his mouth. This was a parent interceding on behalf of a child who was close to death.

Verse 49 tells us that the royal official, expressing his love and pleading prayerfully, said, "Sir, come down before my child die." Jesus replied in verse 50, "You may go, your son will live."

Here we see the royal official took Jesus at His word and departed.

The Bible tells us that while he was still on his way, his servants met him with the news that the boy was living. The royal official asked, "What time did he get better?" They responded, "The fever left him yesterday at the seventh hour (which would have been about 1:00 p.m. that previous day)."

This was the exact same time he spoke with Jesus who told him, "Your son will live."

The noble (royal) official did two things. First, believed what Jesus said immediately, and second, he went. He did not have any doubt. He did not need any signs, and he took Jesus at His word.

Jesus is saying today, "Take me at my word." So many times, we want to see signs, but signs are for unbelievers.

The Bible says in John 4:48, "'Unless you people see signs and wonders,' Jesus told him, 'You will never believe'" (NIV).

The Bible says in Matthew 7:7–8, "Ask, and it shall be given you; seek, and ye shall find; knock, and it shall be opened unto you: For every one that asketh receiveth; and he that seeketh findeth; and to him that knocketh it shall be opened" (KJV).

God cannot and will not lie. There are times when our faith is going to be tested. We see the royal official's faith was being tested. This was an act of faith for him to go without Jesus based on a word.

Sometimes, all you may have is a word. Sometimes, you have to step out on a word. Sometimes, you have to believe God on a word. The words the official had was "You may go, your son will live." The faithful move was when he turned and went back home on a word, trusting Jesus.

How many times did Jesus speak something to you and you did not take Him at His word?

How many times did Jesus speak something to you and you kept saying that you needed confirmation or you were looking for confirmation to come before you would act on the instructions that God gave you?

Yes, Jesus spoke, and He is still speaking. Take Him at His word.

It is done. It is fixed. It is finished. I got this. You are already healed. The finances are there. The way has already been made. The door is opened. The table has been spread. The journey is complete. You did what He instructed you to do. He is pleased. He is not sending you anymore signs.

The Bible says in Matthew 12:39–41, "But he answered and said unto them, An evil and adulterous generation seeketh after a sign; and there shall no sign be given to it, but the sign of the prophet Jonas: For as Jonas was three days and three nights in the whale's belly; so shall the Son of man be three days and three nights in the heart of the earth. The men of Nineveh shall rise in judgment with this generation, and shall condemn it: because they repented at the preaching of Jonas; and, behold, a greater than Jonas is here" (KJV).

Jesus was speaking of the resurrection. Jesus proclaimed here that the Gentiles of Nineveh is more righteous than the Pharisees, because the Gentiles repented but the Pharisees would not take Jesus at His word.

Would you take Jesus at His word today?

TITLE: *"Forgiveness"*

TEXT: Matthew 6:12, 14–15

AUTHOR: Matthew

DATE AND PLACE: The time of writing was considerably after the time of Christ's resurrection (compare 28:15) but obviously before AD 70's destruction of Jerusalem, as predicted in Mathew 24:2. A controversy still exists among scholars as to whether Matthew or Mark was the first Gospel record of the life of Christ.

Biblical Terminology

Forgiveness: Defined by *Holman Bible Dictionary* as an act of God's grace to forget forever and not had people of faith accountable for sins they confess; to a lesser degree the gracious human act of not holding wrong acts against a person.

Blasphemy (*blasphēmĕo* [Greek]): To speak impiously, to speak evil of, defame, or revile. To use speech to bring down another's value, honor, due-respect, or to injure another's reputation in the eyes of others. *Blasphēmĕo* as a verb, according to *Strong's Concordance*, means to "blaspheme, rail at, or revile, and is used in a general way of any contumelious speech, reviling, calumniating, railing at, etc., as of those who railed at Christ."

There are two dimensions of forgiveness.

1. Divine Relationship
2. Human Dimension

Let us first look at the *divine relationship*. Holman notes that divine relationship is the gracious act of God by which believers are put into a right relationship with God and transferred from spiritual death to spiritual life through the sacrifice of Jesus. In the divine dimension, the ongoing gift of God is present. Without this dimension, our lives as Christians would be out of joint and full of guilt.

Second is the *human dimension*. In this dimension, forgiveness is that act and attitude toward those who have wronged us, which restores relationships and fellowships. The first time we see in the Bible where there is a need for forgiveness is in Genesis 3 with Adam and Eve when they disobeyed God and satisfied their own self will. It is noted that this resulted in guilt, loss of fellowship, separation from God, a life of hardship, anxiety, and death, and they lived under the wrath of God.

Forgiveness in Old Testament versus New Testament

When we look at forgiveness as it relates to the Old Testament (OT), the primary means of obtaining forgiveness in the Old Testament was through a sacrificial system of covenant relationship God established when he brought his people out of Egypt. During this system, bringing the sacrifice showed the sense of need. The laying of hands on the living sacrifice symbolized identification of the person with the sacrifice as did releasing the life of the animal through the sacrificial slaughter.

Forgiveness in the New Testament: Jesus is the perfect and final sacrifice through which God's forgiveness is mediated to every person. In the Old Testament, we see only God could forgive sins. However, in the New Testament, Jesus declared that He could. The Bible says in Mark 2:1–12,

> and again He entered Capernaum after *some* days, and it was heard that He was in the house. Immediately many gathered together, so that there was no longer room to receive *them,* not even near the door. And He preached the word to them. Then they came to Him, bringing a paralytic who was carried by four *men.* And when they could not come near Him because of the crowd, they uncovered the roof where He was.

So when they had broken through, they let down the bed on which the paralytic was lying.

When Jesus saw their faith, He said to the paralytic, "Son, your sins are forgiven you."

And some of the scribes were sitting there and reasoning in their hearts, "Why does this *Man* speak blasphemies like this? Who can forgive sins but God alone?"

But immediately, when Jesus perceived in His spirit that they reasoned thus within themselves, He said to them, "Why do you reason about these things in your hearts? Which is easier, to say to the paralytic, '*Your* sins are forgiven you,' or to say, 'Arise, take up your bed and walk'? But that you may know that the Son of Man has power on earth to forgive sins"—He said to the paralytic, "I say to you, arise, take up your bed, and go to your house." Immediately he arose, took up the bed, and went out in the presence of them all, so that all were amazed and glorified God, saying, "We never saw *anything* like this!" (NKJV)

The Bible says in John 8:2–11

Now early in the morning He came again into the temple, and all the people came to Him; and He sat down and taught them. Then the scribes and Pharisees brought to Him a woman caught in adultery. And when they had set her in the midst, they said to Him, "Teacher, this woman was caught in adultery, in the very act. Now Moses, in the law, commanded us that such should be stoned. But what do You say?" This they said, testing Him, that they might have *something* of which to accuse Him. But Jesus stooped down and wrote on the ground with *His* finger, as though He did not hear.

So when they continued asking Him, He raised Himself up and said to them, "He who is without sin among you, let him throw a stone at her first." And again He stooped down and wrote on the ground. Then those who heard *it,* being convicted by *their* conscience, went out one by one, beginning with the oldest *even* to the last. And Jesus was left alone, and the woman standing in the midst. When Jesus had raised Himself up and saw no one but the woman, He said to her, "Woman, where are those accusers of yours? Has no one condemned you?"

She said, "No one, Lord." And Jesus said to her, "Neither do I condemn you; go and sin no more." (NKJV)

Jesus saw His own death as the fulfillment of the Old Testament sacrificial system. Now let us talk about *unforgivable sin.* The sin that is unforgivable is blasphemy against the Spirit.

Remember, *blasphemy* (*blasphēmĕo* [Greek]) means to speak impiously, to speak evil of, defame, or revile; to use speech to bring down another's value, honor, and due-respect; and to injure another's reputation in the eyes of others. *Blasphēmĕo* as a verb, according to *Strong's Concordance,* means to blaspheme, rail at, or revile, and is used in a general way of any contumelious speech, reviling, calumniating, railing at, etc., as of those who railed at Christ.

The Bible says in Matthew 27:39, "Those who passed by were hurling abuse at Him *and* jeering at Him, wagging their heads [in scorn and ridicule]" (Amplified Version).

Those who were passing by were insulting Him with abusive and insolent language, wagging their heads [as a sign of contempt], and saying, "Ha! You who would destroy the temple and rebuild it in [only] three days.
—Mark 15:29 Amplified Version

The Bible says in Luke 22:65, "And they were saying many other [evil and slanderous] things against Him, blaspheming [speaking sacrilegiously and abusively about] Him" (Amplified Version).

And they were saying many other [evil and slanderous] things against Him, blaspheming [speaking sacrilegiously and abusively about] Him.
—Luke 23:39 Amplified Version

Strong noted as to Christ's teaching concerning "blasphemy" against the Holy Spirit in Mathew 12:32: "Whoever speaks a word against the Son of Man will be forgiven; but whoever speaks against the Holy Spirit [by attributing the miracles done by Me to Satan] will not be forgiven, either in this age or in the *age* to come" (Amplified Version).

That anyone with the evidence of the Lord's power before His eyes should declare it to be Satanic, exhibited a condition of heart beyond divine Illumination and therefore hopeless. Divine forgiveness would be inconsistent with the moral nature of God. Accusing Jesus of doing the work of Satan is blasphemy against the Holy Spirit. This is unforgivable.

The Bible says in Mark 3:28–30, "I assure you *and* most solemnly say to you, all sins will be forgiven the sons of men, and all the abusive *and* blasphemous things they say; but whoever blasphemes against the Holy Spirit *and* His power [by attributing the miracles done by Me to Satan] never has forgiveness, but is guilty of an everlasting sin [a sin which is unforgivable in this present age as well as in the age to come]"—[Jesus said this] because the scribes and Pharisees were [attributing His miracles to Satan by] saying, "He has an unclean spirit" (Amplified Version).

> *"I assure you and most solemnly say to you, all sins will be forgiven the sons of men, and all the abusive and blasphemous things they say; but whoever blasphemes against the Holy Spirit and His power [by attributing the miracles done by Me to Satan] never has forgiveness, but is guilty of an everlasting sin [a sin which is unforgivable in this present age as well as in the age to come]"—[Jesus said this] because the scribes and Pharisees were [attributing His miracles to Satan by] saying, "He has an unclean spirit."*
> —Luke 12:10 Amplified Version

The Human Dimension of Forgiveness

The Bible says in Matthew 6:12, 14–15 NKJV, "And forgive us our debts, as we have forgiven our debtors [letting go of both the wrong and the resentment]. For if you forgive others their trespasses [their reckless and willful sins]; your heavenly Father will also forgive you. But if you do not forgive others [nurturing your hurt and anger with the result that it interferes with your relationship with God], then your Father will not forgive your trespasses."

In order to obtain forgiveness from the Lord, we have to also forgive. In the human dimension of forgiveness, there have to be a willingness to forgive others to receive forgiveness.

Let us forgive. Let us be willing to let go of all hurts and wrongs. If you are struggling with unforgiveness, ask God to forgive you for harboring unforgiveness and then help you to be able to forgive.

TITLE: *"Take It to the Lord in Prayer"*

TEXT: 2 Kings 19:14–20 (1 and 2 Kings were originally one book called *Kings* in Hebrew text, from the word in 1:1.

AUTHOR: Unknown. Jewish tradition proposed Jeremiah wrote Kings, which is unlikely because the final event recorded in the book occurred in Babylon in 561 BC. However, Jeremiah never went to Babylon, but to Egypt (Jeremiah 43:1–7). This would also place Jeremiah to be at least eighty-six years old by 561 BC.

DATE AND PLACE: Between 561 and 538 BC

History

We see Hezekiah asked Isaiah to join them in prayer for the remnant that survived, for the remaining who continued to trust the Lord and serve him. Who was Hezekiah? Hezekiah was the king of Judah. He was also the son of Neariah, of the royal family of Judah. The Bible says in 1 Chronicles 3:23 (Revised Version) (British and American—"Hizkiah"), he was an ancestor of Zephaniah (Zephaniah 1:1 KJV, "Hizkiah") as well as one of the returned exiles from Babylon (Ezra 2:16 and Nehemiah 7:21).

Hezekiah was faithful to the Lord. He followed the Lord and obeyed His commands. Hezekiah rebelled against Assyria. Hezekiah's father previously had submitted to Assyria. Hezekiah rebelled against Assyria's control and was independent, and because he did this, it went against the Assyrian rule, and this is where the threat came in. There was to be retaliation.

The commentators stated that Sennacherib succeeded Sargon II as king of Assyria in 705 BC and ruled until 681 BC. Hezekiah rebelled against him by refusing to submit.

McDonald noted that Sennacherib tried to persuade Judah's army not to follow Hezekiah. He also stated that his army was sent against Jerusalem by God. It was at this time Sennacherib warned the people not to believe Hezekiah when he told them that the Lord would deliver. The Assyrians thought that the Lord of Israel was a territorial god like the gods of other nations, and he made claims to be stronger than God.

Hezekiah, in turn, asked Isaiah to join him in prayer for the remnant. Isaiah came with two messages of deliverance from the Lord: "Do not fear," and "The Lord was going to make Sennacherib return home and be destroyed." It was here we see a threatening letter was sent to Hezekiah, reiterating that Hezekiah should not be deceived by God whom they considered to be in the same category as gods of other nations.

Hezekiah took the letter to the temple. It was a common practice to pray when in distress. Hezekiah did spread the letter before the Lord. Hezekiah did something that every one of you have been instructed to do. He casted his cares on the Lord. The Bible says in 1 Peter 5:7, "Casting all your cares upon him; for he careth for you" (KJV).

The Lord heard his prayers. My questions to you today are

1. what is it that has you walking the floors late at night, and
2. what is it that has you so worried that you cannot eat, sleep, or concentrate?

The same way Hezekiah took that letter to the temple and laid it before the Lord, it is time for you to bring that letter. It is time for you to bring that bad doctor's report. It is time for you to bring that eviction notice. Whatever that weight you have been carrying on your shoulders, bring it to the temple. Bring it to the altar and leave it there.

The altar is Jesus. Instead of walking the floor at night over that bad situation, bring it to Jesus. He said, "I am Jehovah Rapha, the Lord that healeth thee." You can bring that doctor's report to Him.

The Bible says in Exodus 15:26, "And said, if thou wilt diligently hearken to the voice of the Lord thy God, and wilt do that which is right in his sight, and wilt give ear to his commandments, and keep all his statutes, I will put none of these diseases upon, thee which I have brought upon the Egyptians for I am the Lord that healeth thee."

I need to inform you that whatever your concern is—wayward children, marital problems, problems on your job, issues with getting that bill passed that you have had sitting on the governor's desk, or that glass ceiling that have been hanging over your head—bring it to Jesus. There is no problem too big or too small.

There is a familiar hymn that we sing quite often in church. It was written in 1855 by Joseph M. Scriven. We sing it, but do we understand how powerful the words of "What a Friend We Have in Jesus" are?

In my closing, it is critical I inform you that there is no problem that is too small. There is no situation that is too hard for God to handle. There is no marriage that is so dead God cannot resurrect it.

The Bible says in John 11:25, "Jesus said unto her, I am the resurrection, and the life; he that believeth in me, though he were dead, yet shall he live."

If Jesus raised Lazarus from the dead, and if He defeated death, Luke 24:1–7 in the Bible says, "Now upon the first day of the week, very early in the morning, they came unto the sepulchre, bringing the spices which they had prepared, and certain others with them. And they found the stone rolled away from the sepulchre. And they entered in, and found not the body of the Lord Jesus. And it came to pass, as they were much perplexed thereabout, behold, two men stood by them in shining garments: And as they were afraid, and bowed down their faces to the earth, they said unto them, Why seek ye the living among the dead? He is not here, but is risen: remember how he spake unto you when he was yet in Galilee, Saying, The Son of man must be delivered into the hands of sinful men, and be crucified, and the third day rise again."

What makes you think your marriage is so dead? What makes you think that your ministry is so dead? What makes you think your dreams are so dead that God cannot resurrect it? No burden is too unbearable, and no financial issue is so pressing that God cannot handle it. God is waiting to talk to you. When you take everything to the Lord, watch those situations begin to dissolve. When you take your mind off those situations and circumstances and focus on Him, magnify Him, and make Him bigger than what it is you are going through, watch God work.

TITLE: *"Lord, Teach Us"*
TEXT: Psalm 90:12–17 (Fourth Book of Psalms)
AUTHOR: Third Prayer of Moses (The Man of God)

Scripture Text

> *So teach us to number our days, that we may apply our*
> *hearts unto wisdom. Return, O Lord, how long? and let*
> *it repent thee concerning thy servants. O satisfy us early*
> *with thy mercy; that we may rejoice and be glad all our*
> *days. Make us glad according to the days wherein thou hast*
> *afflicted us, and the years wherein we have seen evil. Let*
> *thy work appear unto thy servants, and thy glory unto their*
> *children. And let the beauty of the* LORD *our God be upon*
> *us: and establish thou the work of our hands upon us; yea,*
> *the work of our hands establish thou it.*
>
> —Psalm 90:12–17 KJV

Teach us. Instruct us. The Greek word for *teach* is *didáskō*. The usual word for *teach* in the New Testament signifies either to hold a discourse with others in order to instruct them or to deliver a didactic discourse where there may not be direct personal and verbal participation.

To teach means to show or explain how to do something. Lord, teach us how to evaluate the use of time in light of shortness of time. Teach us how to make use of our time. Teach us how to use our time wisely that we may gain a heart of wisdom. Lord, teach us so that we may walk in your way and operate with your wisdom. Lord, teach us to fear you and reverence you.

Lord, teach us the value of time. Teach us to understand the value of spending time with you. Teach us the value of spending time in prayer. Lord, teach us the value of sharing your word with others.

Lord, satisfy us. Meet our expectations early with your mercy. Allow our days of joy to equal our days of distress.

Lord, let your work be seen in your servants and your glory in their children. Let the favor of the Lord rest upon us. Establish the work of our hands. Lord, let what we do by your grace have meaning. Let it be significant. Add value to what we do; and thank you, Lord, for blessing the work of our hands.

TITLE: *"Nevertheless"*

TEXT: Luke 5:4–5

AUTHOR: Luke the Beloved Physician

DATE AND TIME: About AD 52–63 in a Place Unknown

Scripture Text

> *Now when he had left speaking, he said unto Simon, Launch out into the deep, and let down your nets for a draught. And Simon answering said unto him, Master, we have toiled all the night, and have taken nothing: nevertheless at thy word I will let down the net.*
>
> —Luke 5:4–5

When He (Jesus) had stopped speaking, He said to Simon, "Launch out into the deep and let down your nets for a catch." Simon answered and said to Him, "Master, we have toiled all night and caught nothing. Nevertheless, at your word I will let down the net."

Here we see Jesus commanded to let down the nets. He commanded Simon to let the nets down in deep water. Remember, He said to launch out into the deep. To make it simple, for individuals that like to fish, cast your nets out into the deep water. If you would take notice, nets are plural. Simon responded, "Master, we have toiled all night and have caught nothing." This was not making sense to him.

I can imagine Simon saying, "You want me to throw these nets back out here again, Jesus, after I have been out here all night long and the only bite I have gotten was a mosquito bite." I can imagine Simon saying, "Come on, man. You mean you want me to throw these nets back out here again Jesus after I have been out here all night and all I caught was fresh air?"

Simon really did not understand what God was asking him to do. Simon did not understand how God was going to show himself. Simon said, "We have toiled all night and caught nothing. Nevertheless, at your word, I will let down the net." *Nevertheless* is defined as "in spite of that or notwithstanding." What Simon was saying was, "In spite of what I have been through, regardless of not catching anything, at your word Lord, I will let down the net."

After taking a closer look at the text, he only let down one net. When they had done this, the Bible said that they caught a great number. I began to ask God why and He had me to focus on *nevertheless*. Nevertheless at your word.

In other words, at His word, at God's word nevertheless, Simon did not realize what it was that He was speaking. When he said "Nevertheless," he was saying, "Nevertheless, at your word, Lord, I will let down the net." I need to let you know, there is nevertheless with God.

God will always multiply. When you obey God's instructions, God will multiply. The instructions were to launch out into the deep. What are your instructions? What were you waiting for? Nevertheless.

I will bless the Lord at all times. His praise shall continually be in my mouth.

Here we see *I* and *my*—this makes it personal. When David said, "I will bless the Lord at all times," he boasted in the Lord. He gave glory to the Lord. We should also give glory to the Lord, no matter what is going on in our lives or what is going on around us. We should be willing to bless the Lord at all times.

Oh magnify the Lord with me. Let us exalt His name together. Make His name big. Glorify His name. Lift up His name.

Here we see that verses 4–6 deals with the sevenfold testimony of deliverance: "I sought the Lord, and He heard me and delivered me from all of my fears. They looked unto him and were lightened; and their faces were not ashamed. This poor man cried, and the Lord heard him, and saved him out of all his troubles."

Finis Dake pointed out in his commentating that God answered prayers. He delivers from fears. He enlightens His people. Gives his people boldness; saves his people from all troubles and supplies all wants of his people. (Dake, 562).

Again, verses 7–10 mentions the sevenfold promises of deliverance. There is a promise in verse 7: "The angel of the Lord encampeth round about them that fear him and delivereth them."

The next two verses, which are verses 8 and 9, are commands: "Oh taste and see. What it is saying is try the Lord and see. Fear the Lord." That word *fear* is not being afraid of the Lord, but in other words, know him. Learn of him.

Finis Dake notes in verse 10 the promises of Psalm 34:

1. The angel of the Lord encampeth around about them that fear him and delivereth them. (v. 7)

2. There is no want to them that fear Him. (v. 9, Psalm 89:11, and Luke 11:9–11)
3. They that seek the Lord shall not want any good thing. (v. 10 and Matthew 7:11)
4. The eyes of the Lord are upon the righteous and His ears are open to their cry. (v. 10, 15, 17, and John 15:7)
5. The face of the Lord is against them that do evil (v. 16)
6. The righteous cry, and the Lord heareth and delivereth them out of all their trouble. (v. 17)
7. The Lord is nigh unto them that are a broken heart and saveth such as be of a contrite spirit (v. 18)
8. Many are the afflictions of the righteous, but the Lord delivereth him out of them all. (v. 19)
9. Evil shall slay the wicked and they that hate the righteous shall be desolate (v. 21)
10. The Lord redeemeth the soul of His servants and none of them that trust Him shall be desolate (v. 22)

TITLE: *"God Is Light"*

TEXT: 1 John 1:5–10

AUTHOR: Apostle John

DATE AND PLACE: Probably written from Ephesus near the end of the first century. A reasonable date is CAD 90–95. It was likely written to the churches of Asia Minor over which John exercised apostolic leadership.

Apostle John: Who Was He?

1 John is the first and largest in a series of three epistles that bear Apostle John's name. John and James, his older brother, (Acts 12:2) were known as the sons of Zebedee (Matthew 10:2–4). Jesus gave the name sons of thunder (Mark 3:17).

John was one of the three very intimate associates with Jesus, Peter, James, and John. (Matthew 17:1 and 26:37) He was an eyewitness to, and participated in, Jesus's earthly ministry. (1 John 1:1–4) John also identified himself as the disciple whom Jesus loved in the fourth gospel, which he authored.

Here we see that in verse 5, the Bible tells us that God is light.

The message that John and the other apostles preached came from God. Here we see the scriptures start by saying, "This then is the message we have heard from him and declare for you." They spent time with God. They heard from Him. They were not delivering a message that they heard from other men. They delivered what they heard directly from God.

God is light, and in Him is no darkness at all. When we take light and darkness and compare the two:

Light	Darkness
Light represents biblical truth.	Darkness represents error.
Light represents holiness.	Darkness represents falsehood.

Light represents purity.	Darkness represents wrongdoing.
Psalm 119:105: Your word is a lamp to my feet and a light to my path. (Amplified Version)	Romans 13:11–14
Proverbs 6:23	1 Thessalonians 5:4–7
John 1:4 and 8:12	

One thing that the commentator pointed out was that the heretics claimed to be truly enlightened and walking in real light, but John denied it because they did not recognize their sin.

If they did not recognize their sin, it would mean that they had to be spiritually blind. Any time an individual is spiritually blind, they are walking in darkness. Any time an individual is walking outside of Christ, he or she is walking in spiritual darkness.

God is light. God is perfect. God is truth. There is no darkness in Him at all. There is nothing that exists in God's character that affects His truth and holiness. I think something very important was pointed out—if we say we have fellowship with Him, yet we walk in darkness, we lie and do not practice truth. Failure to practice truth, liars, false profession, and sinful walk . . . a true Christian will walk in light and not in darkness. He or she does not operate in falsehood, and the blood of Jesus purifies him from all sin. They constantly walk in light. (2 Corinthians 6:14, Ephesians 5:8, and Colossians 1:12–13) and cleansing from sin constantly occurs.

The Bible says in v. 8 that if we claim to be without sin, we deceive ourselves (self-deception). False teachers not only walk in darkness but also denied the total existence of sin in their lives. When you never admit to being a sinner, salvation cannot take place. (Matthew 19:16–22)

Looking at verses 9 and 10, it tells us that continual confession of sin is an indication of genuine salvation. False teachers do not admit their sin, and this will make Him a liar. God says that all people are sinners. (Psalm 14:3; 51:5; Isaiah 53:6; Jeremiah 17:5–6; Romans 3:10–19, 23; 6:23)

To deny that fact would be to blaspheme God with slander that defames His name.

Sin = Greek: *hamartia*, which means to miss the mark. (1 John 1:7, 8; 3:4, 5, 8, 9; and 5:16, 17)

John speaks of all kind of sin one can recover from and another kind of sin, which one cannot recover from.

The overall teaching of this epistle suggests that those who denied the Christian community to follow heretical antichrist teachings were irrecoverable. Their rebellion and denial of Jesus's true identity leads to unrepentant sin. In the end, their sin produces spiritual death.

The Bible says that we all have sinned (Romans 3:23 and Galatians 3:22), and the penalty for sin is death. But the good news is that God sent Jesus, His only son, to die for us and pay the penalty for our sins (John 3:16 and Romans 5:8). To be saved and to receive everlasting life, we must call upon the name of the Lord Jesus (Acts 2:21 and Romans 10:9–10, 13).

Would you make Jesus Lord? Simply pray this prayer:

> Dear God, I am a sinner. I repent. Would you please forgive me and cleanse me. I believe that Jesus died for my sins. I believe that you raised Him from the dead. Thank you for sending Jesus to die for me.
>
> Jesus, I ask you to come into my heart and be my Lord. Baptize me with your Holy Spirit. I receive everlasting life.
>
> Amen. Welcome to the body of Christ.

TITLE: *"Destined to Win"*

SUBTOPIC: You Are an Overcomer

TEXT: John 15:18–19

AUTHOR: John (The Beloved Disciple)

DATE AND PLACE: About AD 90 in a place unknown

Scripture

> *If the world hate you, ye know that it hated me before it hated you. If ye were of the world, the world would love his own: but because ye are not of the world, but I have chosen you out of the world, therefore the world hateth you.*
>
> —John 15:18–19

Definitions

Overcomer: an overcomer is defined by *Webster* as a person who prevails in spite of opposition, difficulties, or weaknesses. A person who defeats someone or something in a conflict or a struggle. Greek: *nikaō*—to subdue, overcome, conquer, prevail, or get the victory.

Destined: bound for a certain destination, ordained, appointed, or predetermined to be or do something.

Here we see in John 15:18–19 that Jesus is having a discussion with His disciples. He also informs them that the world stands convicted. Not only is He informing them, but He is also reminding His disciples: "Hey the world hates you."

You are not a part of this world.

The NIV puts it like this:

> *If the world hates you, ye know that it hated me before it hated you. If ye were of the world, the world would love his*

own: but because ye are not of the world, but I have chosen
you out of the world, therefore the world hateth you.

—John 15:18–19

You are chosen. I need to remind you, not only are you chosen but you are also an overcomer; and because you are an overcomer, you are destined to win. You are a king's kid. It is very important that you know and understand that.

The commentator pointed out that while His disciples are to love each other, they would be hated and treated as enemies by the world. The world is that evil system whose head is Satan and whose agents are in opposition to Jesus and His cause.

Finis Dake also noted that this is the Thirty-Sixth New Testament prophecy here in John 15:18–21 that is fulfilled and is being fulfilled.

With Christ telling His disciples, "If ye were of the world, the world would love his own: but because ye are not of the world, but I have chosen you out of the world, therefore the world hateth you." (It is noted that Christ testified this of His disciples three times here in verse 19 and 17:14–16)

Dake also noted that the reasons why the world hated Jesus are

1. the world hates reproof (John 3:19);
2. Christian living exposes the evil of the world (Romans 12:2 and Titus 2:11–12);
3. the Christian light exposes darkness in the world (Philippians 2:15 and John 3:18–20);
4. the world is blind (2 Corinthians 4:4);
5. Christians are not of the world (John 15:19 and 17:14–16);
6. the world is at war with Christians (John 16:33, Ephesians 6:12, and 1 John 5:4);
7. the world has enmity against God (James 4:4 and Matthew 18:7);
8. Christians hate the ways of the world (1 John 2:15–17);
9. Christians live separate from the world (James 1:27, Romans 12:2, and 2 Peter 2:20);

10. the world is ignorant concerning Christianity (Galatians 2:20 and 2Corinthaians 5:17);
11. the world is ignorant of God (John 15:21);
12. and Jesus predicted it (John 15:18–21).

All of this was done out of ignorance. The world lacked knowledge of the relationship between the Father and Jesus. Jesus was informing them of what was to come. The world's hatred of Jesus and rejection of His teaching had been openly expressed in persecution. However, what I need you to focus on is not the world's hatred and not the persecution. Your focus is to be on who you are and to whose you are.

I need to remind you that you belong to God. You have been chosen, and you do not belong to this world.

The Bible says in 1 Peter 2:9, "But ye are a chosen generation, a royal priesthood, an holy nation, a peculiar people; that ye should shew forth the praises of him who hath called you out of darkness into his marvelous light" (KJV).

You are an overcomer. Your job is to continue to please God. The Bible says in Proverbs 16:7, "When a man's ways please the Lord, he maketh even his enemies to be at peace with him" (KJV).

Do not worry about the persecution because persecution must come. Your focus is to remain not on pleasing the Lord. Why? You are destined to win. It does not matter what situation or circumstance that may arise, just know that God has already made a way. You have been ordained to win. You have the victory. You can praise Him for the victory. Even if it looks like you are losing, you are still winning.

My husband, the late great elder Willie M. Richardson Jr., told me about a runner he was watching on YouTube, and he said, "I do not understand how this girl won after running out of her shoe." I went back and pulled up the story. Her father is a boxer. She is age seven. She was running in a race. She lost her shoe and fell behind, but despite that, she still won. The commentator said that if you can get anything from this story, never give up. I told Elder Richardson that when God has His hand on your life, you are destined to win.

She was destined to win. It did not matter that she ran out of her shoe. That was her race to win.

I am reminded of the story of the turtle and the rabbit (hare) in the race (you know the story), and the rabbit started running fast. The turtle was moving at a slow pace. The rabbit ran, singing and laughing because the turtle was so slow, but the turtle kept his pace. The rabbit knew he was going to win because the turtle was so slow. The rabbit decided to stop and took a nap. When the rabbit finally woke up, he started back running and made it to the finish line. When he got to the finish line, the turtle was there, waiting for him.

It does not matter where you start. It does not matter how fast you run. Just keep running and do not stop. Keep trusting God. You are destined to win. Do not pull over to fight. Do not pull over to address foolishness. Do not pull over to chase rumors. Set your pace and keep it moving. Keep looking straight ahead. Do not look to the left or to the right. Just keep running. You are destined to win.

I do not like to close without an open invitation to salvation. The Bible says we all have sinned (Romans 3:23 and Galatians 3:22), and the penalty for sin is death. But the good news is that God sent Jesus, His only son, to die for us and pay the penalty for our sins (John 3:16 and Romans 5:8). To be saved and to receive everlasting life, we must call upon the name of the Lord Jesus (Acts 2:21 and Romans 10:9–10, 13)

Would you make Jesus the Lord? Simply pray this prayer:

> Dear God, I am a sinner. I repent. Would you please forgive me and cleanse me. I believe that Jesus died for my sins. I believe that you raised Him from the dead. Thank you for sending Jesus to die for me.
>
> Jesus, I ask you to come into my heart and be my Lord. Baptize me with your Holy Spirit. I receive everlasting life.
>
> Amen. Welcome to the body of Christ.

TITLE: *"Touch Not My Anointed and Do My Prophet No Harm"*

TEXT: Numbers 12:1–16 and 1 Chronicles 16:22

AUTHOR: MOSES IS THE AUTHOR OF NUMBERS. 1 CHRONICLES: Isaiah and Ezra or Final compilers using public records of the Nation of Israel. Among the records were Nathan, Gad, Iddo, Ahijah, Jehu, and others

DATE AND PLACE: Numbers was written by Jordan near Jericho in 1490 BC in the plains of Moab, just before entrance into Canaan. 1 Chronicles was written in Palestine 1279–461 BC by scribes and prophets whose duty was to record events during the time of whatever king or kings they served under.

History

Here we see in Numbers 12:1–16 that this particular chapter deals with the rebellion of Aaron and Miriam who opposed Moses. Miriam and Aaron were the older sister and brother of Moses. They spake against Moses out of jealousy because of the cushite (Ethiopian) wife that Moses married by the name of Zipporah. Miriam was a prophetess. She was in the position of first rank among the women of Israel. The Bible says in Exodus 15:20–21, "And Miriam the prophetess, the sister of Aaron, took a timbrel in her hand; and all the women went out after her with timbrels and with dances. And Miriam answered them, Sing ye to the LORD, for he hath triumphed gloriously; the horse and his rider hath he thrown into the sea."

One thing that Finis Dake pointed out is that being a sister of two chief men, she caused rebellion because she thought she was being supplanted by a foreigner. Jethro had brought the wife and sons of Moses from Midian to Sinai in order to reunite the family, and he gave advice to Moses. Moses was invited by his father-in-law and brother-in-law to go along with them to be leaders in showing them the best places to camp. It displeased Miriam to see the new comers given such attention, and her resentment was shared by Aaron.

The two of them challenged the right of Moses to serve as the leader of the whole nation, but Miriam seemed to have been the chief instigator of this ungodliness because the punishment fell on her alone. Aaron was simply misled by his sister, as he did previously when he allowed the people to urge him to sin and build the golden calf.

My question to you today is, Who is in your ear? Moses married one of the descendants of the son of Abraham. Here we see that during the conversation that took place between Miriam and Aaron, there were two questions asked:

1. Hath the Lord indeed spoken only by Moses?
2. Hath He not spoken also by us?

In other words, Is our brother Moses the only person God speaks to or the only person God uses? Can God not use us also?

They had an anointing. Their anointing, as pointed out, was to judge and govern, not to prophesy. They had a different anointing on their life. The Bible says that the Lord heard it.

My brothers and my sisters, do not fool yourselves or let anyone fool you into thinking that when engaging into conversations about God's anointed, His chosen vessels, even if they are not physically in your presence, that God is not aware of what is going on. The Bible says that God heard it.

My brothers and my sisters, don't you know that as God's chosen vessels, you do not have to defend yourselves all of the time? There are some times when God will defend you, and He will do it suddenly.

Verse 3 reminds us that Moses was very meek above all the men upon the face of the earth. God spake suddenly unto Moses and unto Aaron and Miriam. The Lord came down in a pillar of the cloud, and He said, "Hear now my words."

The Bible says in Numbers 12:6–9, "And he said, Hear now my words: If there be a prophet among you, I the Lord will make myself known unto him in a vision, and will speak unto him in a dream. My servant Moses is not so, who is faithful in all mine house. With him will I speak mouth to mouth, even apparently, and not in dark speeches; and the similitude of the Lord shall he behold: wherefore then were ye not afraid to speak against my servant Moses? And the anger of the Lord was kindled against them; and he departed" (KJV).

Now we see that when the cloud departed, Miriam became leprous, white as snow. Aaron, after seeing what happened to Miriam, begged Moses for mercy. He said, "I beseech thee, lay not this sin upon us."

Beseech: to beg for urgently or anxiously, to request earnestly, or to make supplication.

Aaron realized where they had sinned and he confessed. He was able to admit that he sinned. Then and only then, after Miriam and Aaron spake against Moses, we see that Miriam became leprous.

The Bible says in 1 Chronicles 16:22, "Saying, Touch not mine anointed, and do my prophets no harm" (KJV).

Do not be fooled into thinking that you could speak against God's anointed and for God not to hear it. Do not be fooled into thinking that you could raise your hand against God's anointed and for God not to see it. Do not be tricked by the enemy into thinking that you could lay traps and snares against God's chosen vessels and for God not to see it. I must also warn you that God's anointed vessel is not just clergy. God has His hands on lay people. He has his hands on those that are sitting in the pews. They don't have to wear a clergy collar to be God's anointed.

Be careful who is in your ear this season. Be careful who solicits you to do their dirty work this season because it will likely be a boomerang. Keep your hands and your mouth off God's chosen vessels. If you do not understand what God is doing in a person's life or ministry, then just pray for them, but keep your mouth and hands off them.

Are you saved? I do not like to close without an open invitation to salvation. The Bible says we all have sinned (Romans 3:23 and Galatians 3:22), and the penalty for sin is death. But the good news is that God sent Jesus, His only son, to die for us and pay the penalty for our sins (John 3:16 and Romans 5:8). To be saved and to receive everlasting life, we must call upon the name of the Lord Jesus (Acts 2:21 and Romans 10:9–10, 13)

Would you make Jesus Lord? Simply pray this prayer:

> Dear God, I am a sinner. I repent. Would you please forgive me and cleanse me. I believe that Jesus died for my sins. I believe that you raised Him from the dead. Thank you for sending Jesus to die for me.

> Jesus, I ask you to come into my heart and be my Lord. Baptize me with your Holy Spirit. I receive everlasting life.

> Amen. Welcome to the body of Christ.

TITLE: *"It Rains on the Just and the Unjust"*

TEXT: Matthew 5:43–48 (Key Verse 45)

AUTHOR: Matthew (meaning "gift of the Lord" was the other name of Levi, the tax collector who left everything to follow Christ)

DATE AND PLACE: This gospel was written at a relatively early date prior to the destruction of the temple in AD 70. Some scholars have proposed a date as early as AD 50.

Scripture

> *You have heard that it was said, "You shall love your neighbor (fellow man) and hate your enemy." But I say to you, love [that is, unselfishly seek the best or higher good for] your enemies and pray for those who persecute you so that you may [show yourselves to] be the children of your Father who is in heaven; for He makes His sun rise on those who are evil and on those who are good, and makes the rain fall on the righteous [those who are morally upright] and the unrighteous [the unrepentant, those who oppose Him]. For if you love [only] those who love you, what reward do you have? Do not even the tax collectors do that? And if you greet only your brothers [wishing them God's blessing and peace], what more [than others] are you doing? Do not even the Gentiles [who do not know the Lord] do that? You, therefore, will be perfect [growing into spiritual maturity both in mind and character, actively integrating godly values into your daily life], as your heavenly Father is perfect.*
>
> —Matthew 5:43–48 Amplified Version

He makes His sun rise on the evil and on the good, and sends rain on the just and on the unjust. He—the Bible is referring to God Almighty—God makes His sun to rise. Only God can make the sun rise and only God can make the sun set. God makes the sun to rise and set on the evil as well as the good, on the righteous as well as the unrighteous. It is God's decision to make, not man's decision, as to how He is going to send rain, where He is going to send rain, and when He is going to send rain. It is also God's decision as to what types of rain He is going to send. Yes, I said what types of rain He is going to allow to fall.

There are two types of rain that we are going to talk about today.

1. Physical Rain: water falling in drops, condensed from vapor in the atmosphere
2. Spiritual Rain: showers of blessings, sometimes, spiritual storm

However, in the end, God can decide to send rain on the just or the unjust. That is why it is important to always have an umbrella at all times.

1. Physical umbrella
2. Spiritual umbrella

The *physical umbrella* is a collapsible shade for protection against weather, consisting of fabric stretched over hinged ribs radiating from a central pole.

The *spiritual umbrella* is God—the ultimate umbrella. He protects us from everything. You have to have a relationship with God and obey His commands, honor His authority, and obey His word. Under this umbrella, God establishes a structure: family (husband and parents, Ephesians 5:21–29; 6:1–4, and Colossians 3:18–21); government leaders (Romans 13:1, Titus 3:1, and 1 Peter 2:13–17); church leaders, elders, and other believers (Hebrews 13:7, 17; 1 Peter 5:5; and Ephesians 5:21); and employers (1 Peter 2:18, Titus 2:9, Ephesians 6:5, Colossians 3:22, and 1 Timothy 6:1–2).

Definitely have on your armor. Remember the sun if it is raining, because the sun will shine again. The Bible says that He makes His sun rise on evil and the good, and sends rain on the just and on the unjust.

Just: based on or behaving according to what is morally right and fair.

Unjust: not based on or behaving according to what is morally right and fair.

Example 1: Recently, we had rain here in Sumter. On the north side, it poured. As I drove on Broad Street, it also rained. However, it did not rain as hard. Just because it was not raining as hard, that does not mean that the people on the north side of town did something bad nor are bad people because it rained hard at that particular time.

Example 2: Last week, while it rained in South Carolina, Texas, and other parts of the United States had very bad weather, snow, power outages, loss of water, pipes breaking in their homes, and even loss of lives. That does not mean that the people of Texas are bad people or the citizens of South Carolina are better than the citizens of Texas.

I hear you asking the question, What does this have to do with this message? I am glad that you asked. The Bible says in verse 43, "You have heard that it was said, you shall love your neighbor and hate your enemy, but I say to you, [in other words, this is Jesus talking], love your enemies. Bless those who curse you, do good to those who had you, and pray for those who spitefully use you and persecute you that you may be sons of your father in heaven."

For it is He, it is God, who makes the sun rise on evil and the good. He has the power. Yeah, I know everyone is telling you and whispering in your ear, "Man, if I were you, I wouldn't have anything to do with that joker." Well, they are not you.

I know the law of retribution says An Eye for an Eye. I know you want to keep your status with your friends. I know you want to keep your reputation of being hard. I know you are trying to go along to get along. I know you have gotten used to having lots and lots of people around you telling you just how great you are and telling you what you want to hear. Notice, I said what you want to hear. Yeah, I know that people keep telling you this and that but I (Jesus) say to you:

Love your enemies. I see what they did, and what they did was not done to you. You are going off what you heard. I know their works the same way I know your works, and I say, "Love your enemies." I see how you were dogged out in the past. However, that is in the past. Now I am saying, "Let it go and love your enemies." I see how they have cursed you and dragged your name through the mud, but I say, "Bless them that curse you." I know that they smile in your face, but inside, they harbor hate. I see how they treat you on your job. I see how your name went across the manager's desk for promotions but got swept under the rug. I see how when it is time for invitations to parties, weddings, showers, and other engagements, your name is left off the list. Jesus said, "I allowed it." God designed you that you would not fit in. You were trying to fit into places where He did not call you to fit in.

He allowed them to think that something was wrong with you. He allowed them to think that you were dysfunctional. He allowed them to drop you so the right person could pick you up. He allowed you to be rejected, only for a season. He just needed you to pray for those who spitefully used you and persecuted you.

The whole time you were thinking there was something wrong with you, there is nothing wrong with you. There is nothing wrong with them. God was just opening your eyes. He was preparing you for the rain. God wants you to love. He is teaching you how to love unconditionally. God is getting you to see things, people, situations, and circumstances from His perspective. God wants you to love everyone, regardless of what season they find themselves in. It is God who allows it to rain. Whether he rains down blessings or allows the storms to rage, it is God who has the power to control it. Everything moves by the power of God.

Rainy days are coming. It is time to let go of some stuff and grip the solid rock. On Christ the solid rock I stand, all other ground is sinking sand. Stop listening to what others say and stand on the Word of God. Jesus said, "But I say, to love your enemies. Bless those who curse you and do good to those who hate you. Pray for those who spitefully use you and persecute you. Love, bless, pray for, and do good to all."

Retribution is the Mosaic law. Let it go. An eye for an eye is not what God wants. If you kill my dog, I'll kill your cat. That is not what God wants you to do. Let it go. Ask God to teach you how to love.

For those who have weathered the storm, you have endured hardship, you loved your enemies, you blessed those who cursed you, and you prayed for those who despitefully used you and persecuted you. It is getting ready to rain. God is getting ready to shower down blessings.

TITLE: *"Saving the Best for Last"*

TEXT: John 2:1–10

AUTHOR: John

DATE AND PLACE: It was probably written in the '90s of the first century.

Here we see the Bible telling us in chapter 2 verse 1 that on the third day, there was a wedding in Cana of Galilee. This wedding was to take place on the third day after Jesus left Jordan to start His ministry. The marriage feasts in those days were not like the marriages we are accustomed to today. During that time, marriage feasts lasted, sometimes, a week. This specific marriage feast was in Cana, located on a low hill on the side of a rich upland plain about seven miles north of Nazareth.

Mary (the mother of Jesus), as well as some of Jesus's disciples, attended this wedding feast. (The text was not clear as to how many of Jesus's disciples attended.) While attending this marriage feast, something happened. They ran out of wine. This would have been a very embarrassing moment, but Mary told Jesus, "They have not wine."

There were many things I could imagine that Jesus could have done, but Jesus, being the loving and merciful person that he is, responded and said, "Woman, what have I to do with thee? My hour has not yet come." He knew it was not yet His time. He did not disrespect His mother. In other words, He was saying, "I have nothing to do with this matter. It is not time for me to perform miracles yet." He did not go and tell everyone, "Look they are out of wine." He did find amusement in this. He was serious. This was a serious occasion.

Mary, knowing who Jesus was, remembered when she was told about whom she had to birth into the world. The Bible says in Matthew 1:21, "And she shall bring forth a son, and thou shalt call his name Jesus: for he shall save his people from their sins" (KJV).

Surely, if Jesus could save His people from their sins, He could perform a miracle and create some more wine. The last recorded words of Mary were these words, as she looked to the servants, in verse 5, "Whatever he says to you, do it."

The Bible says that there were six water pots of stone, according to the manner of purification of the Jews, containing twenty to thirty gallons a piece. Jesus instructed them to fill the water pots with water. Six of those water pots would have held about 162 gallons, making more than 2,400 servings.

I am not sure, and the text is not clear as to when exactly the water was turned into wine. I am not sure if it turned into wine when they filled the pots with water. I am not sure if the water turned into wine as they drew it out. I am not sure if the water turned into wine as the master tasted it. That really is not that important. The most important factor is that the miracle did take place. The water was turned into wine. Jesus turned it into wine, and because Jesus turned it into wine, it was authentic. Because Jesus turned into wine, it was as if it had aged. Because Jesus turned it into wine, it was the best.

When Jesus does something, it is always good. The master pointed out that every man at the beginning sets out the good wine. When every man have drunk, then the inferior you have kept the good wine until now. You have saved the best for last.

That is the same thing that God is doing with you. Yeah, I know you thought you were being held back, but God is just saving the best for last.

God had to show me through a revelation of carpenter bees coming in our sanctuary. I sprayed the bee on Sunday. The bee laid in the window on Sunday and Monday, and on Tuesday, the maintenance man knocked him on the floor, because I left it there so the maintenance people could identify the bee. When the trustee went to pick it up on the hand fan, the bee was still alive.

I was talking to my brother about it, and he said, "You know, the bee was in the church, praying." Then I thought about it. God will allow even your enemy to spray you, and He will still keep you. God is keeping us alive in the midst of a deadly situation. When folks spray you, when folks try to kill you, even when they write you off, I need to let you know that it is God who is preserving you. He is saving the best for last. Do not worry. Do not fret. I know it looks like God have forgotten about you. I know it looks like God did not hear your prayer. But God is getting ready to perform a miracle in your situation. He is saving the best for last.

TITLE: *"If I Be Lifted Up"*

TEXT: John 12:32

AUTHOR: Apostle John

DATE AND PLACE: Uncertain, probably during the late first century

Scripture

> *And I, if I be lifted up from the earth, will draw all men unto me.*
>
> —John 12:32 KJV

Jesus: Who is He?

Jesus was born in the last years of the reign of Herod the Great who died (4 BC) as recorded in Josephus. His parents are Mary and Joseph. He was conceived between betrothal and wedding. His conception was through the Holy Spirit. His mother was still a virgin. His birth was at Bethlehem. He was brought up in Nazareth. His father, Joseph, is said in Matthew 13:55 to have been a carpenter. Jesus is also said to have been a carpenter in Mark 6:3. It is presumed that Jesus received the education of the devout poor in Israel, with thorough instruction in the Hebrew scripture. His public career began when he left home for the Jordan River to be baptized by John the Baptist.

John 3:22 and 4:1 tells us that for a time, it appears that Jesus conducted a ministry of baptizing parallel to that of John the Baptist.

After John the Baptist's arrest (Mark 1:14), Jesus embarked upon a new kind of ministry. His message of the kingdom acquired a new urgency. As a result, the temptation (Mark 1:12–13), which included a vision of God's victory over Satan (Luke 10:18).

Jesus moved from baptizing and went to synagogues for a time. He then spoke in open air. He reached out to the people instead of waiting for them to come to Him. However, He continued preaching the coming of the kingdom.

Michael Coogan pointed out that Jesus never defined what He meant by the kingdom, but it means God's coming in saving power and strength, defeating the powers of evil and inaugurating salvation for Israel.

Jesus was recognized as a rabbi and teacher.

There are differences between Jesus's teachings and the teachings of the Pharisees. Jesus emphasizes more strongly than the Pharisees that God demands not just outward conformity to the law, but the whole person, not just love of neighbor, but love of enemy. (Matthew 5:21–48)

For Jesus, God's demand is summed up in the double commandment of love.

Jesus's prophetic preaching presupposes His wisdom preaching.

God's coming in His kingly rule is an act of mercy and forgiveness (an important aspect of Jesus's message). (Mark 2:5, Luke 4:47, and Matthew 18:23–35)

Jesus's preaching of repentance is connected with his offer of forgiveness. (Mark 1:15; 6:12; and Mathew 11:20)

Jesus brought no new teachings about God.

Jesus appeared as a charismatic healer as well as a preacher and teacher.

Jesus performed exorcisms, which He claimed were the action of the spirit (Matthew) or finger (Luke) of God. To deny this spirit at work in His exorcism was blasphemy, a sin for which there would be no forgiveness (Mark 3:29). Thus, both healings and exorcisms were related to His message.

Jesus celebrated meals with the outcast.

At one point, He broke off his Galilean ministry and transferred his activities to Jerusalem.

He fed the multitudes. (Mark 6:30–52; 8:1–9; 13; and John 6:1–71)

Jesus continued to preach and teach in Jerusalem, as He had done in Galilee.

He engaged in conflicts with His adversaries. His enemies engaged Him on specific issues seeking to entrap Him into self-incrimination.

He engaged in theological conflict with religious authorities in Jerusalem.

Jesus's challenge reached its climax when He entered Jerusalem and cleansed the temple.

John 11:47–53 tells us about the Sanhedrin meeting. The Sanhedrin decided to get rid of Jesus out of fear of any disturbance of the peace would lead to Roman intervention and destroy the delicate balance between Jewish and Roman powers.

On the eve of Passover, Jesus celebrated a farewell meal with His disciples.

After supper, Jesus and his disciples went out to the Garden of Gethsemane (Mark 14:32 and John 18:1) where he was arrested.

The Trials of Jesus

- **First Trial** (John 18:13–23) was held before Caiaphas's father-in-law, Annas, who was the high priest during that year.
- **Second Trial** (Matthew 26:57–68, Mark 14:53–65, and John 18:24) was held before Caiaphas and the Sanhedrin. On accusations that Jesus claimed to be the Messiah, the Son of God, this was considered to be blaspheme and worthy of death.
- **Third trial** (Mark 15:1a and Luke 22:66–71) was held before Sanhedrin (ruling body of seventy men in Israel). Jesus was declared guilty of blasphemy. He was sent to Roman officials because they did not have authority to carry out capital punishment. When Rome took over Judea and began direct rule through a prefect in AD 6 capital jurisdiction, the right to execute was taken away from the Jews and was given to the Roman governor.
- **Fourth Trial** (Matthew 27:11–14, Mark 15:1b–5, Luke 23:1–7, and John 18:28–38) was held before Pilate (governor of Judea) on accusations of treason. He was found to be innocent. Jesus was mistreated and mocked.
- **Final Trial** (Matthew 27:15–26, Mark 15:6 and 15, Luke 23:18–23, and John 18:39–19:16) was held before Pilate on

accusations of treason. Pilate tried to remove himself of guilt. He left the decision to the mob, giving them a choice of Jesus or Barabbas. Pilate washed his hands and allowed Jesus to be crucified.

And I, if I be lifted up from the earth, will draw all men unto me.

—John 12:32

Jesus already knew His purpose. He predicted His death in verse 23.

And Jesus answered them, saying the hour has come that the Son of Man should be glorified. This hour was the crucifixion, which would pay the price for Adam's fallen race.

In order for the Son of Man to be glorified, which guarantees the resurrection, Jesus could not be glorified unless He was resurrected. He had to die in order to be resurrected.

Jesus tells us in verse 32, "And if I be lifted up from the Earth (on the Cross) will draw all men unto me. This cross is where the victory is."

Everybody who comes to Jesus now, believing in what he did, trusting in the finished work of Jesus Christ, and His atoning death, will be saved.

Starts Talking about a Capable Wife

- A wife, who is also a mother, shall rejoice in time to come.
- Honor, better, dignity—she shall rejoice in time to come.
- She smiles at the future.
- She has no anxiety.
- Her family is well taken care of.
- She is energetic.
- She is well occupied.
- The key to her character is her spiritual life.
- She is a woman who fears the Lord. In other words, she is a woman who has a relationship with the Lord.

- Her spiritual house is in order.
- She is a woman of valor.
- She is a woman of strength.
- She is a woman of great character and integrity.
- She works late into the night (now this working late does not necessarily mean on a man's job. She is working in her home. She is taking care of her home. She is taking care of her children. She is taking care of the things that God has assigned to her hands.)
- She is a seamstress we know, because verse 24 tells us that she makes linen garments and sells them. She is also a businesswoman because she sells them.
- She is up in the night working, but she is working from home.

- ▪ This is a woman who manages her household with discretion and speaks wisdom

- She is a woman who is strong and resilient and serves her family.
- She inspires kindness and perseverance in her children.
- She serves her family well, and she will earn the eternal gratitude of her children and her spouse.
- She started out in the beginning as a capable wife.
- Because of the path that she has treaded, she is a virtuous woman.

TITLE: *"Get Your House in Order for Jesus Is Soon to Come Back"*

TEXT: 2 Kings 20:1–11

AUTHOR: Unknown, possibly Jeremiah or a group of prophets

Who Was Hezekiah?

- Hezekiah was the son of Ahaz, King of Judah.
- He became king at the age of twenty-five.
- He reigned in Jerusalem for twenty-nine years.
- His mother's name was Abijah, the daughter of Zechariah.

The Bible said that he did what was right in the eyes of the Lord, just as his father, David.

- He removed high places.
- He smashed sacred stones.
- Cut down Ashera poles (sacred poles).
- He broke into pieces the bronze snake that Moses made (the Israelites had been burning incense to it and called it Nehushtan—Hebrew for bronze, snake, unclean thing).

The bronze snake was made to cure the Israelites of the venomous snakes (Numbers 21:4–9.) It demonstrated God's presence and power, and it reminded the people of God's mercy and forgiveness. However, they turned it into an idol and began to worship it.

We have to be careful of who and what we are worshipping. God wants us to worship Him and Him alone.

Here we see that Hezekiah trusted the Lord. The Bible says there was no one like him among all the kings of Judah before or after him. The Lord was with him and he was successful in whatever he undertook. However, the Bible said that Hezekiah became ill to the point of death. I don't know what kind of illness he had because the text did not say. The text did say that the Lord sent the prophet Isaiah (the eagle eye prophet) to tell him to put his house in order because he was not going to recover.

So many people are walking around in this world today that has become sick to the point of death. They have become sick physically. They have become sick spiritually. People in our churches have become sick physically and spiritually. People in our communities have become sick physically and spiritually. People in our nation have become sick physically and spiritually. People in this world have become sick physically and spiritually.

When I prayed, I asked the Lord to give me a word for the nation, and he told me, "Put your house in order because I am coming back one day." When this message was given to Hezekiah, he turned his face to the wall and prayed to the Lord. He reminded God of how he walked before Him faithfully and done what was good in His eyes, and he wept.

Keep in mind, it was stated that in Judah's history of a hundred-year period, Hezekiah was the only faithful king.

The Lord did respond to Hezekiah's prayer.

I need to let someone know that the Lord did not respond to Hezekiah's prayer because of Hezekiah being so great, nor did he respond to Hezekiah's prayer because he felt sorry for Hezekiah. He did not respond to Hezekiah's prayer because of his pedigree. He did not respond to Hezekiah's prayer because of how much money he had or because of his educational background.

It was because of Hezekiah's faith and prayers that got God's attention.

The same way the Lord spoke back then, He is still speaking that way today. Set your house in order, your spiritual house, because Jesus is coming back one day. If you keep going like you are going, you are going to die.

John 15:5 NIV says, "I am the vine; you are the branches, if a man remains in me and I in him, he will bear much frit. Apart from me you can do nothing. If anyone does not remain in me, he is like a branch that is thrown away and withers; such branches are picked up, thrown into the fire and burned."

Hezekiah prayed, reminded God of his faithfulness, and he wept. Hezekiah turned his face to the wall.

The Lord sent the same prophet back to Hezekiah and told him, "I heard your prayers on the third day. From now, you will go up to the temple of the Lord, and I will add fifteen years to your life, and I will deliver you and this city from the king of Assyria."

He was instructed to prepare a poultice of figs.

Put your house in order and listen for God's instructions.

It is time for us to put our houses in order for healing to take place.

- spiritual healing to place
- for our children's healing to take place
- healing to take place in the land
- healing to take place in our homes
- healing to take place in our finances

If my people, who are called by my name, will humble themselves and pray and seek my face and turn from their wicked ways, then will I hear from heaven and will forgive their sin and will heal their land.

—2 Chronicles 7:14 NIV

> *For all have sinned and fall short of the glory of God.*
> —Romans 3:23 KJV

This means everyone, (everyone was placed in the same category. There was no separation or division of men) all have sinned and fell short of the glory of God.

> *But Scripture has locked up everything under the control of sin, so that what was promised, being given through faith in Jesus Christ, might be given to those who believe.*
> —Galatians 3:22 KJV

The law could not give eternal life, it could only give death, which was and is its exact penalty. Eternal life comes by faith in the promise. Eternal life comes by faith in Jesus Christ and what He did on the cross. There have to be belief in what Jesus Christ did on the cross.

> *Therefore, just as sin entered the world through one man, and death through sin, and in this way death came to all people, because all sinned—.*
> —Romans 5: 12 NIV

This man that the scripture is talking about is Adam, and the death that it is speaking of is both spiritual as well as physical death.

> *For the wages of sin is death, but the gift of God is eternal life in Christ Jesus our Lord.*
> —Romans 6:23 NIV

This death is spiritual death. Spiritual death separates individuals from God. Eternal life is gained by that which Christ did on the cross. Our faith has to be in what Jesus did on the cross.

> *For God so loved the world that he gave his one and only Son, that whoever believes in him shall not perish but have eternal life.*
>
> —John 3:16 NIV

God loved the world with an unconditional love. God gave His son to die on the cross to redeem humanity.

> *But God demonstrates his own love for us in this: While we were still sinners, Christ died for us.*
>
> —Romans 5:8 NIV

Jesus died for all; he died for those that loved Him as well as those that hated him. His death for all humanity showed his unconditional love.

> *And everyone who calls on the name of the Lord will be saved.*
>
> —Acts 2:21 NIV

This is for everyone, not just certain people.

> *If you declare with your mouth, "Jesus is Lord," and believe in your heart that God raised him from the dead, you will be saved. For it is with your heart that you believe and are justified, and it is with your mouth that you profess your faith and are saved. For, "Everyone who calls on the name of the Lord will be saved."*
>
> —Romans 10:9–10, 13 NIV

Why Not Make Jesus Lord?

- The Bible says we all have sinned (Romans 3:23 and Galatians 3:22), and the penalty for sin is death (Romans 5:12 and 6:23).
- But the good news is that God sent Jesus, His only Son, to die for us and pay the penalty for our sins (John 3:16 and Romans 5:8).
- To be saved and to receive everlasting life, we must call upon the name of the Lord Jesus (Acts 2:21 and Romans 10:9–10, 13)

Prayer of Salvation

Dear, God, I come to you in the name of Jesus. I admit that I have sinned. I ask you to forgive me and cleanse me. Thank you for sending Your Son to die for me.

Jesus, I ask you to be my Savior and Lord. I receive everlasting life. Thank you for saving me. Amen.

Sources

Dake, Finis Jennings. 1991. *Dake's Annotated Reference Bible.* Dake Bible Sales.

Institute of Basic Life Principles. https://iblp.org/.

MacDonald, William. 1980. *Believer's Bible Commentary.* Thompson Nelson.

Nelson's Three-in-One Bible Reference Companion. 1982. Thompson Nelson.

The New International Webster's Standard Dictionary. 2006. Trident Reference.

Thompson Chain-Reference Bible: King James Version. n.d. B.B. Kirkbride Bible.

Thompson Chain-Reference Bible: New International Version. 1982. B.B. Kirkbride Bible.

Author's Publications

Woman of Change	ISBN 978-1-4349-9720-3
Cooking Made Simple	ISBN 978-1-6270-9308-4
Gourmet Cuisine, Venison Cooking	ISBN 13: 978-1-6300-4059-8
Chicken/Turkey: "Ya Gotta Love It"	(hardback) 978-1-5434-5355-3
	(paperback) 978-1-5434-5356-0
	(e-book) 978-1-5434-5357-7
Sermons	(print) 978-1-9845-2958-9, 1984529587
	(eText) 978-1-9845-2957-2, 1984529579
The Armor of God	(hardback) 978-1-7960-5686-0
	(paperback) 978-1-7960-5685-3
	(e-book) 978-1-7960-5684-6
Jonah	(hardback) 978-1-6641-2489-9
	(paperback) 978-1-6641-2488-2
	(e-book) 978-1-6641-2487-5

Author's Songs

"Reign Jesus Reign"
"A Melody for Jesus"
"Yes Jesus, Yes Lord"
"We Shall Behold the Name of the Lord"
"Every Time I Turn Around"
"I Love You Lord"

Index

A

Aaron, 30–32
Abijah (mother of Hezekiah), 48
Adam, 9, 51
adultery, 10
Ahaz (king of Judah), 48
altar. *See* Jesus
Annas (high priest), 44
anointed vessels, 31–32
anointing, 31
Antipas, Herod, 5
Ashera poles, 48
Assyria, 14

B

Babylon, 14
beseech, 5, 32
Bethlehem, 42
blasphemy, 8, 10–12, 43–44
blind, spiritually, 24

C

Caiaphas (high priest), 44
Cana, 5, 39
Capernaum, 5
Coogan, Michael, 43

D

Dakes, Finis, 5, 21, 27, 30
darkness, 23
David (forefather of Hezekiah), 21, 48
death, 3, 5–6, 9, 11, 25, 29, 32, 44–45,
    48–49, 51–53
    atoning, 45

deliverance, testimony of, 21
destined, 26
didáskō. *See* teach
disciples, 23, 26–27
divine forgiveness, 12
divine relationship, 8

E

erotao. *See* beseech
eternal life, 51–52
everlasting life, 25, 29, 33, 53
evil system, 27
exorcisms, 43
Ezra, 1, 30

F

faith, 6–8, 10, 51–52
false teachers, 24
fear, 21
forgiveness, 8–9, 11, 13

G

Galilee, 5–6, 16, 43
Garden of Gethsemane, 44
Gentiles, 7
God, 7, 16, 19, 21, 23–24, 34–37, 40–41
    unconditional love of, 52
    See also Jesus

H

hamartia. *See* sins
healing, 43, 50
Hezekiah (king of Judah), 14–15,
    48–50
holiday seasons, of 2020, 3

Holman Bible Dictionary, 8
human dimension, 9, 13

I

Isaiah (prophet), 14–15, 30, 49
Israel, 43
Israelites, 48

J

James (John's brother), 23
Jehovah Rapha. *See* Jesus
Jeremiah, 14
Jerusalem, 1, 8, 14, 43
Jesus, 6–7, 9–11, 15–16, 19, 26, 39–40,
    42, 45, 49, 52
    reasons why the world hated, 27
    teachings of, 43
    trials of, 44
John (apostle), 23
John the Baptist, 42
Jonas (prophet), 7
Jordan River, 42
Joseph (father of Jesus), 42
Judaea, 5–6
just, 35

L

laws, 1, 51
    Mosaic, 38
    of Moses, 1, 10
    of retribution, 36, 38
Lazarus, 16
letter, threatening, 15
light, 23
Lord, joy of the, 1–2
Lord of Israel, 14. *See also* Jesus
love, 6, 26–27, 34, 36–38, 43, 52, 59

M

marriage feasts, 39

Mary (mother of Jesus), 39–40, 42
merimnao, 3
miracles, of Jesus, 5–7, 12–13, 39–41
Miriam (sister of Moses), 30–32
Moab, 30
Moses, 30–31

N

Nazareth, 42
Neariah (father of Hezekiah), 14
Nehemiah (cupbearer), 1
Nehushtan. *See* snake, bronze
nevertheless, 20
nikaō. *See* overcomer
nobleman, 5–6

O

1 John, 23
overcomer, 26

P

pandemic, 3–4
Paul (apostle), 3
Pharisees, 7, 43
physical umbrella, 35
Pilate, 44
Pilate (governor of Judea), 44
prayers, 3–4, 14–15, 17, 25, 29, 33,
    49, 53
promises, 21–22

R

rabbit, 29
rain, physical, 35
rebellion, 30
Richardson, Willie M., Jr., 28
Rome, 44
runner, 28

S

sacrificial system, 9, 11
salvation, 24, 29, 32, 52
Sanhedrin meeting, 44
Sargon II (king of Assyria), 14
scribes, 1, 10
Scriven, Joseph M., 16
    "What a Friend We Have in Jesus," 16
Sennacherib, 14–15
Simon (fisherman), 19–20
sins, 8, 10–13, 24–25, 29, 31–32, 43, 51, 53
snake, bronze, 48
spiritual darkness, 24
spiritual death, 8, 25, 52
spiritual rain, 35
spiritual umbrella, 35
Strong's Concordance, 5, 8, 11
supplication, 4

T

teach, 17
turtle, 29

U

unjust, 36

W

water gate, 1
wedding, 37, 39
"What a Friend We Have in Jesus" (Scriven), 16
wife, capable, 46–47

Z

Zebedee (fisherman), 23
Zechariah (father of Abijah), 48
Zephaniah (prophet), 14
Zipporah (wife of Moses), 30

www.ingramcontent.com/pod-product-compliance
Lightning Source LLC
Chambersburg PA
CBHW031156250726
48655CB00002B/994